Organic Perfumes:

35 Recipes of 100% Organic and Non-Toxic Perfumes + Bonus Fresh Deo Recipes

Table of content:

Introduction

Organic perfumes are based on natural botanical oils, such as absolutes and essential oils. People are moving toward do-it-yourself natural perfumes instead of expensive perfumes available in stores. Commercial perfumes may have chemicals, and these can be harmful to your sensitive skin. Organic perfumes are free from harmful chemicals, and you can wear these natural fragrances without any problem. These perfumes are beneficial for your health. All the fragrances and scents in the perfume will be natural instead of synthetic.

For instance, your organic jasmine perfume will surely have jasmine, but the perfume available in the store may not have jasmine. It may contain a few real flowers of jasmine, but most of the scent may come from synthetic aromas produced in the laboratory. People are frequently opting for organic perfumes to get the following advantages:

- Get rid of allergic reactions because there are no chemicals in the natural perfume.

- These perfumes will not irritate your skin because organic perfumes are free from alcohol.

- Essential oils are beneficial for your skin.

- These are good for your environment because of zero chemicals and harmful ingredients.

- Organic perfumes are cheap and easy to prepare at home.

These are small advantages of organic perfumes, and there are various recipes available for your assistance. Alcohol is a common ingredient in perfumes, but it can irritate your skin and stain your cloth. The organic ingredients are utilized in the natural perfumes and may not irritate your skin. You can use flowers and essential oils to make organic perfumes. Some perfumes may be extracted from fruits. These products are better than products filled with chemicals. You can use natural ingredients to make organic perfumes and deodorants.

In this book, you will learn to make organic perfumes, and there are 30 organic recipes for 100% Toxic Free Divine Smelling Perfumes.

Chapter 1 – Toxic Free Divine Smelling Perfumes

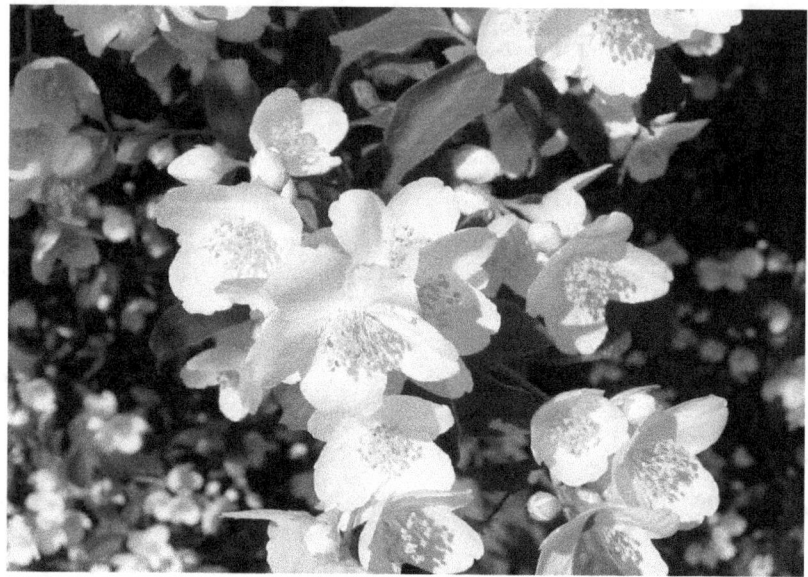

There are a few recipes that will help you to make Toxic Free Divine Smelling Perfumes at your own home. These recipes are easy to follow for everyone:

Recipe 01: Jasmine Perfume

- Jojoba Oil: 2 tablespoons

- Distilled water: 1 tablespoon

- Jasmine: 30 drops

- Vanilla: 5 drops

- Lavender: 5 drops

Directions:

Mix all essential oils in one glass bottle and keep this bottle aside for almost two days. Mix in distilled water and shake them well. Leave this blend for nearly four weeks in one dark and cool spot. In the case of any sediment, you can strain this mixture through a cheese cloth. Pour it in a spray bottle and enjoy.

Recipe 02: Natural Perfume

- Jojoba Oil: 1 oz

- Distilled water: 1 oz

- Jasmine oil: 5 drops

- Lemon oil: 3 drops

- Orange oil: 3 drops

- Sandalwood oil: 3 drops

Directions:

Combine all ingredients in one small container and mix them well by tipping the bottle up and down. You can apply it on the neck, behind your ear or wrist. It will keep you fresh and fragrant for almost 2 to 3 hours.

Recipe 03: Rose Petal Perfume

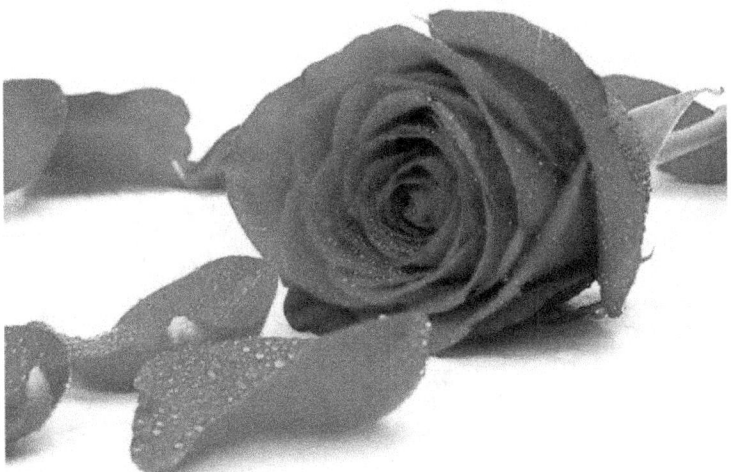

You will need almost 30 – 35 petals of rose with strong fragrance.

Put these petals in one cup and fill this cup with water to soak all petals. Strain this water, but secure these rose petals. Put them in pastel-and-mortar and mash these petals to grind them.

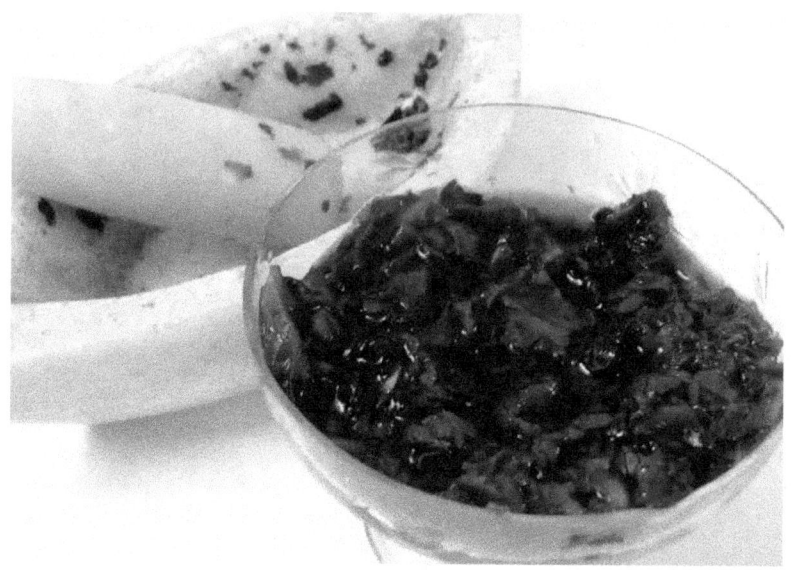

Put these grind petals in strained water and once again strain moisture from petals. Continue this procedure until the water becomes brownish-pinkish-orangish color. Now take out all rose petals and enjoy this rose water. You can put it in a spray bottle.

Recipe 04: Organic Flower Perfume

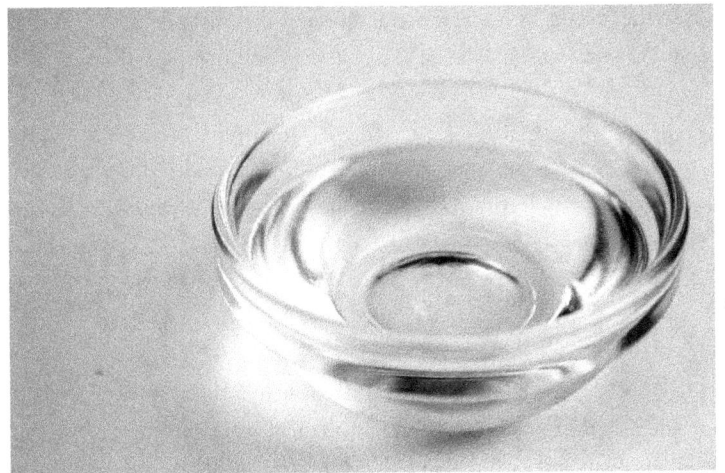

- Chopped flowers: 1 1/2 cups

- Glass bowl with lid

- Cheesecloth

- Small saucepan

- Distilled water: 2 cups

- Sterilize a glass bottle with airtight cap

Directions:

You can take the petals of your favorite flower and wash them to remove sediment and dirt with water.

You have to soak flowers and put cheesecloth in the bowl with edges. The cheesecloth should overlap the bowl. You can put flowers in the cheesecloth-lined bowl and carefully pour water on petals to cover these flowers. Cover this bowl with one lid and place this bowl aside for one night.

In the next day, remove the lid of the bowl and slowly join the four corners of the cheesecloth and lift the pouch of flowers from this water bowl. Squeeze this pouch on the saucepan and extract scented water. Simmer this water on low heat until only one teaspoon liquid left.

Put this perfume in the bottle and secure its cap. This fragrance can be used for one month. You should secure it in a dark and cold place.

Recipe 05: Lavender Scent

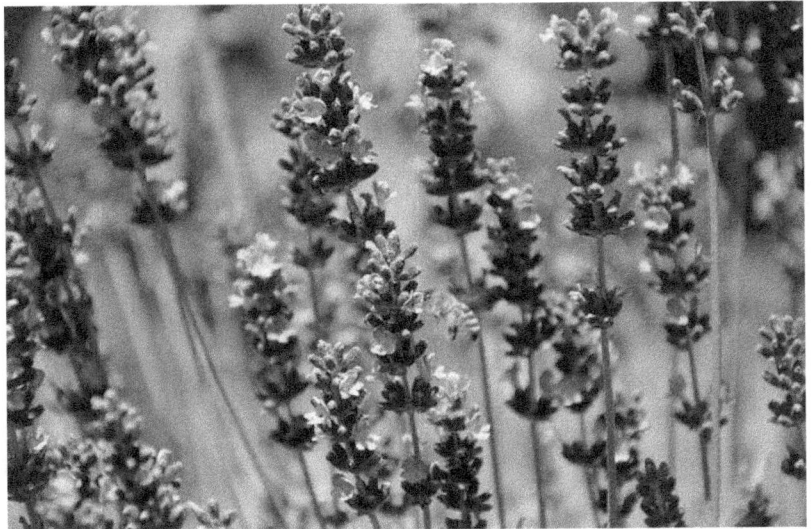

- Distilled Water

- Plastic Bottle

- 3 Lavender flower and 1 red rose

- Eye dropper

Directions:

Remove buds and petals from rose and lavender flowers. Wash all flower petals to remove mud. Add petals in the cooking pan in the boiling water and reduce heat to let it simmer. After 15 minutes, pour this water along with buds and petals in a jug to cool down.

Now use cheesecloth to strain scented water, and throw petals and buds. The water will be turned pink in color and the petals should be white. You can use an eye dropper or pipette to transfer this perfume to a perfume atomizer. The perfume is ready to use.

Recipe 06: Fragrance of Rose and Clove

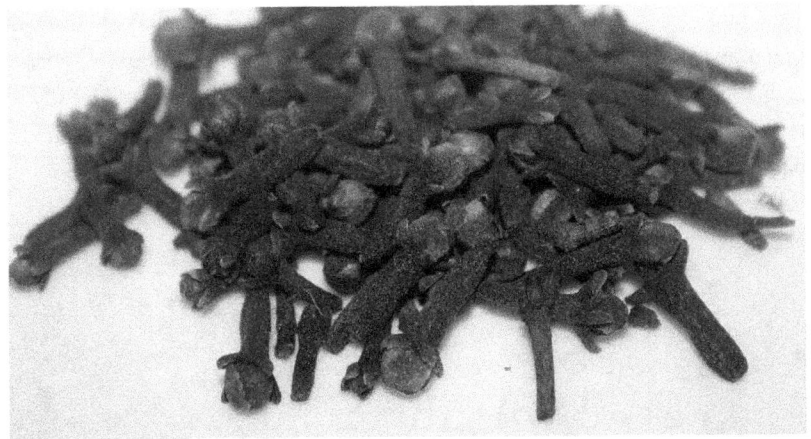

- Jojoba oil: 1/4 cup

- Clove oil: 2 to 3 drops

- Rose oil: 1 teaspoon

- Dark glass bottle

Directions:

Take one dark bottle to because it is good to secure your perfume. Blend all ingredients (except clove) and mix them well. You can pour this mixture at least 12 hours. Clove can overpower other ingredients; therefore, you can add it in the last and pour one drop at one time. Select a cool and dry area to store it. You can dab it on pulse points to enjoy the long-lasting fragrance. You can increase the amount of rose oil to make the scent strong.

Recipe 07: Orange and Mint Cologne

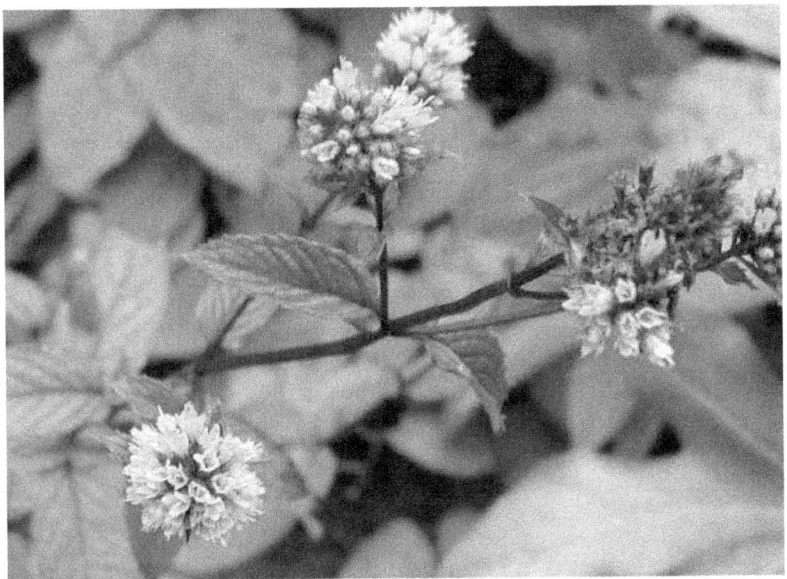

- Orange peel (remove white pith): 1 orange

- Mint leaves: a handful

- Sweet citrus EO (essential oil): 5 drops

- Peppermint EO: 1 drop

- Vodka (optional)

Directions:

Take a clean mason jar and combine mint and orange peel in one Mason jar. Pour vodka or distilled water in the jar and put the lid back. Shake this jar well and leave for almost 4 to 6 weeks. The cologne is ready, and now you can add sweet citrus and peppermint in one cup of cologne. You can pour this blend in one spray bottle for later use.

Chapter 2 – Organic Perfumes with Flowers and Essential Oil

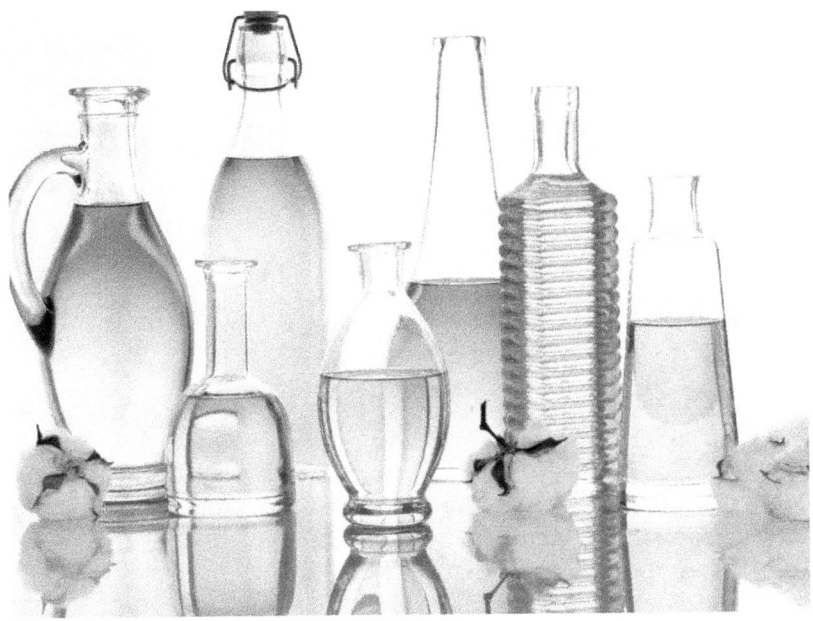

There are some essential oils that prove good to make organic perfumes. These perfumes are good for your skin.

Recipe 08: Romantic Perfume

- Cedarwood EO: 3 drops

- Bergamot EO: 15 drops

- Sandalwood: 3 drops

- 100 proof vodka (optional): 300ml

- 2 drops vanilla EO

Directions:

First add vodka (if using) in one jar and put all the ingredients and shake them well. It will be good to secure this mixture in a dark bottle and put this bottle in one dark and cool place for almost 7 days. You can rub it on your pulse points to enjoy the enduring fragrance.

Recipe 09: Sandalwood Perfume

- Water (distilled): 2 cups

- Perpetual essential oil: 5 drops

- 100 Proof vodka: 3 tablespoons

- Sandalwood EO: 10 drops

- Peony EO: 10 drops

Directions:

In the first step, add vodka (if using) in one jar and put all the ingredients and shake them well. It will be good to secure this mixture in a dark bottle and put this bottle in one dark and cold place for almost seven days. You can rub it on your pulse points to enjoy the enduring fragrance.

Recipe 10: Mesmerizing Blend

- Water (distilled): 2 cups

- Sandalwood EO: 5 drops

- Vodka or Grape fruit EO: 3 tablespoons

- Cassis EO: 10 drops

- Bergamot EO: 10 drops

Directions:

In the first step, add vodka (if using) in one jar and put all the ingredients and shake them well. It will be good to secure this mixture in a dark bottle and put this bottle in one dark and cold place for almost seven days. You can rub it on your pulse points to enjoy the enduring fragrance.

Recipe 11: Lilly Aromatic Oil

- Lilly flowers: 12

- Sweet almond EO: 20 drops

Directions:

Take a jar and put oil and lily flowers in this jar. Cover this jar and put aside for almost 24 hours. You can use a wooden spoon to press down flowers to release their fragrance. After 24 hours, you can use funnel to strain flowers. If you want strong scent, you can increase flowers and infusion time. Seal this jar to keep it away from sunlight. You can use this oil as massage or bath oil.

Recipe 12: Extract Rose Water at Home

- Fresh roses: 2 (1 cup petals)

- Distilled water: 2 cups

- Vodka (it is optional): 1 teaspoon

Directions:

You should have fresh roses and wash them properly to remove any insects and pesticides. Put these petals in the saucepan and soak in distilled water. It is time to add vodka and cover the pan with its lid and keep it on low heat. There is no need to let them boil or simmer because it can ruin the actual properties of rose. Wait for almost 20 minutes, until the water change its color. It is time to strain this liquid in a mason jar and close its lid. This jar can be stored in your refrigerator for almost seven days.

Recipe 13: Chamomile Bled

- Water (distilled): 2 cups

- Rose oil: 5 drops

- Valerian oil: 10 drops

- Chamomile oil: 10 drops

- Body glitter (as per need)

Directions:

In the first step, take one jar and put all the ingredients and shake them well. It will be good to secure this mixture in a dark bottle and put this bottle in one dark and cold place for almost seven days. You can rub it on your pulse points to enjoy the enduring fragrance.

Recipe 14: Rosemary Perfume

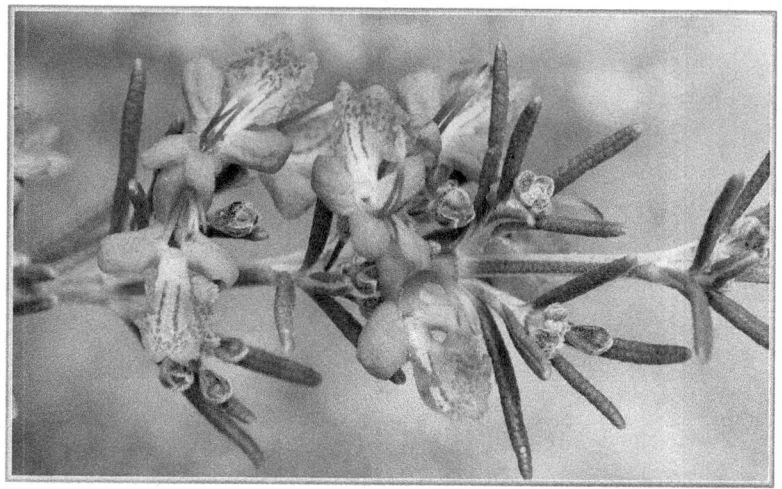

- Water (distilled): 2 cups

- Hypericum EO: 5 drops

- Rosemary EO: 10 drops

- Cypress EO: 10 drops

- Vodka (optional): 3 tablespoons

Directions:

In the first step, add vodka (if using) in one jar and put all the ingredients and shake them well. It will be good to secure this mixture in a dark bottle and put this bottle in one dark and cold place for almost seven days. You can rub it on your pulse points to enjoy the enduring fragrance.

Recipe 15: Misty Perfume

- Ylang-ylang EO: 2 drops

- Passionflower EO: 3 drops

- Neroli EO: 3 drops

- Vodka (optional): 1/2 part (300ml)

Directions:

In the first step, add vodka (if using) in one jar and put all the ingredients and shake them well. It will be good to secure this mixture in a dark bottle and put this bottle in one dark and cold place for almost seven days. You can rub it on your pulse points to enjoy the enduring fragrance.

Recipe 16: Bergamot Perfume

- Water (distilled): 2 cups

- Sandalwood EO: 5 drops

- Vodka (optional): 3 tablespoons

- Cassis rose oil: 10 drops

- Bergamot EO: 10 drops

Direction:

In the first step, add vodka (if using) in one jar and put all the ingredients and shake them well. It will be good to secure this mixture in a dark bottle and put this bottle in one dark and cold place for almost seven days. You can rub it on your pulse points to enjoy the enduring fragrance.

Recipe 17: Good Night Perfume

- Musk EO (organic): 4 drops

- Sandalwood EO: 4 drops

- Jojoba oil: 2 teaspoons

- Frankincense EO: 3 drops

Directions:

In the first step, add vodka (if using) in one jar and put all the ingredients and shake them well. It will be good to secure this mixture in a dark bottle and put this bottle in one dark and cold place for almost seven days. You can rub it on your pulse points to enjoy the enduring fragrance.

Chapter 3 – Solid Perfumes for Him and Her

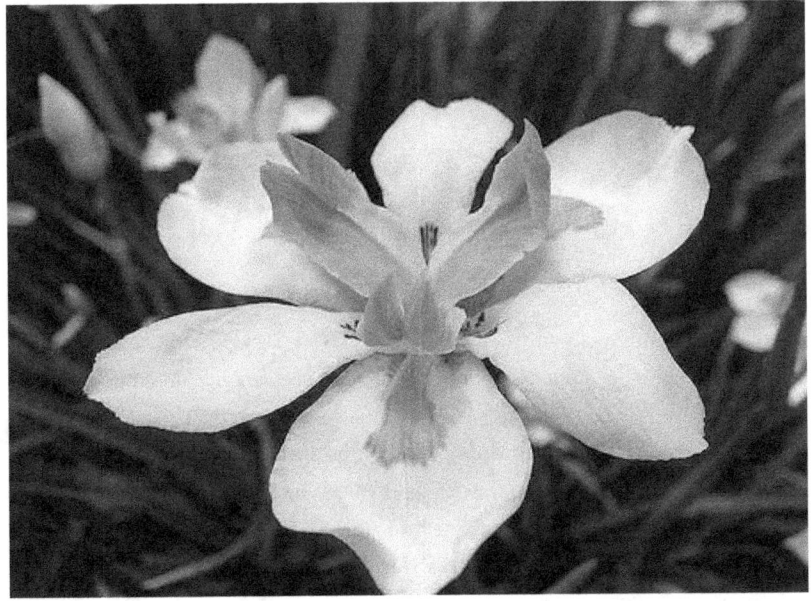

If you want solid perfumes, there are a few recipes to make your own solid perfumes. These solid blends will be great for everyone:

Recipe 18: Jasmine Fragrance

- Fresh Jasmine flowers: 1 medium bowl

- Moisturizing cream

Directions:

You can use any moisturizing cream as per your skin. Take a wide jar and cover it with a thick layer of cream (the pot should be wide enough to put your hand comfortably in this pot. Fill the jar with flowers and cover each corner of this jar with flowers. Secure the lid and keep it for almost one month. It is important to regularly change the jasmine flowers and throw old one in dustbin. After one month, you can check the jar and smell this cream. If the fragrance is strong, you can remove flowers and mix this cream with other cream for later use.

Recipe 19: Solid Perfume

- Grapefruit EO: 17 drops

- Ginger EO: 14 drops

- Beeswax pastilles: 1 tablespoon

- Vetiver essential oil: 10 drops

Directions:

Use microwave or double boiler to melt the beeswax. It is time to mix all essential oils in the beeswax. You have to pour this mixture in one jar or bottle. It is easy to pour solid perfume in a heart-shaped or round locket to keep it always with you.

Recipe 20: Almond Oil Solid Perfume

- Beeswax: 1 tablespoon

- Almond oil: 1 tablespoon

- Glass container: 1

- Straw: 1

- Pyrex bowl or glass jar for mixing: 1

- Saucepan: 1

- Orange EO: 6 drops

- Ylang-ylang EO: 4 drops

- Bergamot oil: 4 drops

- Rosewood EO: 3 drops

- Frankincense oil: 3 drops

- Jasmine oil: 2 drops

Directions:

Collect ingredients and supplies before starting you work. Measure out almond oil and wax in the glass jar. Put one inch water in a saucepan and place the bowl or jar containing wax in this water. Let this water boil to gradually melt wax.

Once the wax turn into liquid, you can remove it from heat. Mix in essential oils in the wax with a stirring stick because the wax will turn into solid. Pour this liquid wax in the container immediately before it turns into solid. It may take almost 30 minutes to let it cool.

Just rub your finger on the surface of wax and apply it behind your ears and in your wrists.

Recipe 21: Jasmine Solid Perfume

- Beeswax: 1 tablespoon

- Almond oil: 1 tablespoon

- Glass container: 1

- Straw: 1

- Pyrex bowl or glass jar for mixing: 1

- Saucepan: 1

- Jasmine EO: 5 drops

- Rose EO: 4 drops

- Ylang-ylang EO: 2 drops

- Cedar EO: 2 drops

Directions:

Collect ingredients and supplies before starting you work. Measure out almond oil and wax in the glass jar. Put one inch water in a saucepan and place the bowl or jar containing wax in this water. Let this water boil to gradually melt wax.

Once the wax turn into liquid, you can remove it from heat. Mix in essential oils in the wax with a stirring stick because the wax will turn into solid. Pour this liquid wax in the container immediately before it turns into solid. It may take almost 30 minutes to let it cool.

Just rub your finger on the surface of wax and apply it behind your ears and in your wrists.

Recipe 22: Loveswept Solid Bar

- Almond oil: 2 tablespoons

- Beeswax: 2 tablespoons

- Jasmine EO: 2 to 4 drops

- Clove EO: 2 drops

- Vanilla Extract: 2 drops

Directions:

Collect ingredients and supplies before starting you work. Measure out almond oil and wax in the glass jar. Put one inch water in a saucepan and place the bowl or jar containing wax in this water. Let this water boil to gradually melt wax.

Once the wax turn into liquid, you can remove it from heat. Mix in essential oils in the wax with a stirring stick because the wax will turn into solid. Pour this liquid wax in the container immediately before it turns into solid. It may take almost 30 minutes to let it cool.

Just rub your finger on the surface of wax and apply it behind your ears and in your wrists.

Recipe 23: Sandalwood Perfume

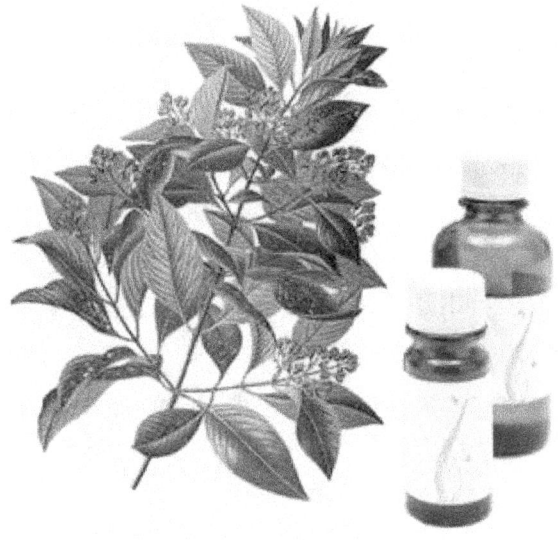

- Beeswax: 1 tablespoon

- Almond oil: 1 tablespoon

- Glass container: 1

- Straw: 1

- Pyrex bowl or glass jar for mixing: 1

- Saucepan: 1

- Jasmine EO: 5 drops

- Rose EO: 4 drops

- Sandalwood EO: 2 drops

- Cedar EO: 2 drops

Directions:

Collect ingredients and supplies before starting you work. Measure out almond oil and wax in the glass jar. Put one inch water in a saucepan and place the bowl or jar containing wax in this water. Let this water boil to gradually melt wax.

Once the wax turn into liquid, you can remove it from heat. Mix in essential oils in the wax with a stirring stick because the wax will turn into solid. Pour this liquid wax in the container immediately before it turns into solid. It may take almost 30 minutes to let it cool.

Just rub your finger on the surface of wax and apply it behind your ears and in your wrists.

Recipe 24: Fruity Perfume

- 35 drops grapefruit EO

- 15 drops orange EO

- 1 tablespoon beeswax pastilles

- 10 drops Vetiver essential oil

- 5 drops roman chamomile EO

- 10 drops Clary Sage EO

Directions:

Collect ingredients and supplies before starting you work. Measure out almond oil and wax in the glass jar. Put one inch water in a saucepan and place the bowl or jar containing wax in this water. Let this water boil to gradually melt wax.

Once the wax turn into liquid, you can remove it from heat. Mix in essential oils in the wax with a stirring stick because the wax will turn into solid. Pour this liquid wax in the container immediately before it turns into solid. It may take almost 30 minutes to let it cool.

Just rub your finger on the surface of wax and apply it behind your ears and in your wrists.

Recipe 25: Earthen Scent

- 20 drops lavender EO

- 14 drops cedarwood EO

- 1 tablespoon beeswax pastilles

- 30 drops marjoram essential oil

- 3 drops ylang-ylang EO

Direction:

Use microwave or double boiler to melt the beeswax. It is time to mix all essential oils in the beeswax. You have to pour this mixture in one jar or bottle. It is easy to pour solid perfume in a heart-shaped or round locket to keep it always with you.

Chapter 4 – Amazing All-natural Perfumes

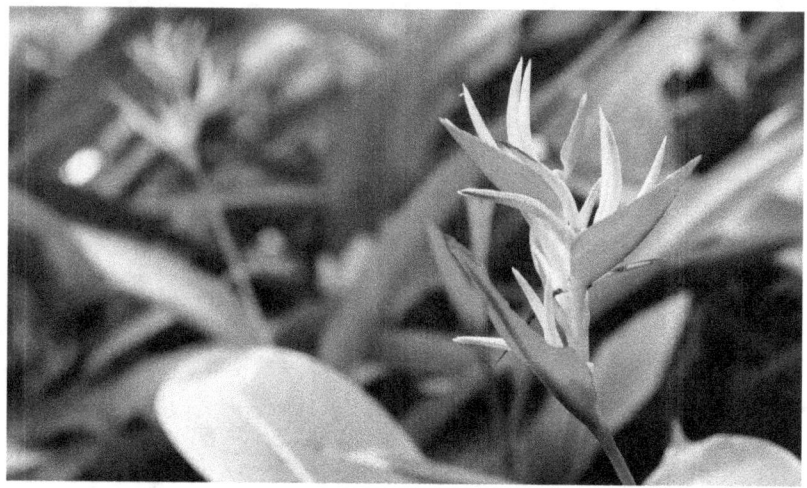

If you want natural perfumes with unique ingredients, you can get the advantage of these recipes.

Recipe 26: Chocolate Scented Blend

- Water (distilled): 2 cups

- Perpetual essential oil: 5 drops

- 100 Proof vodka: 3 tablespoons

- Vanilla EO: 10 drops

- Cocoa EO: 10 drops

Directions:

In the first step, add vodka (if using) in one jar and put all the ingredients and shake them well. It will be good to secure this mixture in a dark bottle and put this bottle in one dark and cold place for almost seven days. You can rub it on your pulse points to enjoy the enduring fragrance.

Recipe 27: Lemon and Orange Blend

- 2 cups water (distilled)

- 5 drops perpetual essential oil

- 3 tablespoons 100 Proof vodka

- 10 drops Orange EO

- 10 drops Lemon EO

Directions:

In the first step, add vodka (if using) in one jar and put all the ingredients and shake them well. It will be good to secure this mixture in a dark bottle and put this bottle in one dark and cold place for almost seven days. You can rub it on your pulse points to enjoy the enduring fragrance.

Recipe 28: Peppermint and Lemon Blend

- 2 cups water (distilled)

- 5 drops peppermint essential oil

- 3 tablespoons 100 Proof vodka (Optional)

- 10 drops sandalwood EO

- 10 drops Rose EO

Directions:

In the first step, add vodka (if using) in one jar and put all the ingredients and shake them well. It will be good to secure this mixture in a dark bottle and put this bottle in one dark and cold place for almost seven days. You can rub it on your pulse points to enjoy the enduring fragrance.

Recipe 29: Apricot Perfume

- 2 cups water (distilled)

- 5 drops perpetual essential oil

- 3 tablespoons Almond oil or Vodka

- 10 drops apricot EO

- 10 drops Sandalwood EO

Directions:

In the first step, add vodka (if using) in one jar and put all the ingredients and shake them well. It will be good to secure this mixture in a dark bottle and put this bottle in one dark and cold place for almost seven days. You can rub it on your pulse points to enjoy the enduring fragrance.

Recipe 30: Cinnamon Perfume

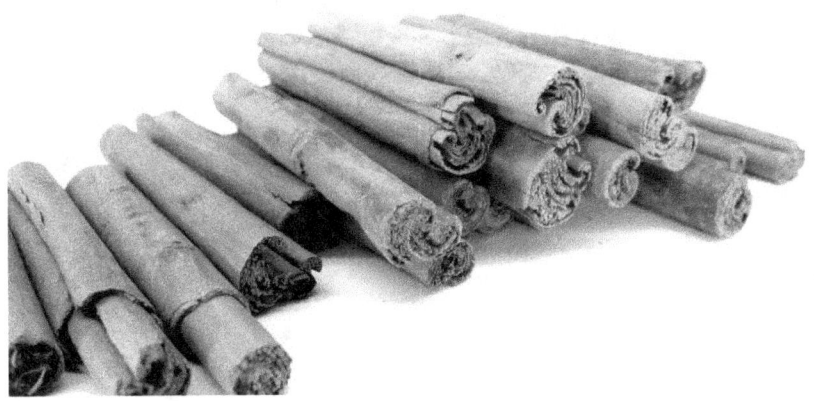

- Water (distilled): 2 cups

- Cinnamon essential oil: 5 drops

- 100 Proof vodka or Almond Oil: 3 tablespoons

- Sandalwood EO: 10 drops

- Neem EO: 10 drops

Directions:

In the first step, add vodka (if using) in one jar and put all the ingredients and shake them well. It will be good to secure this mixture in a dark bottle and put this bottle in one dark and cold place for almost seven days. You can rub it on your pulse points to enjoy the enduring fragrance.

Chapter 5 – Deodorant Recipes

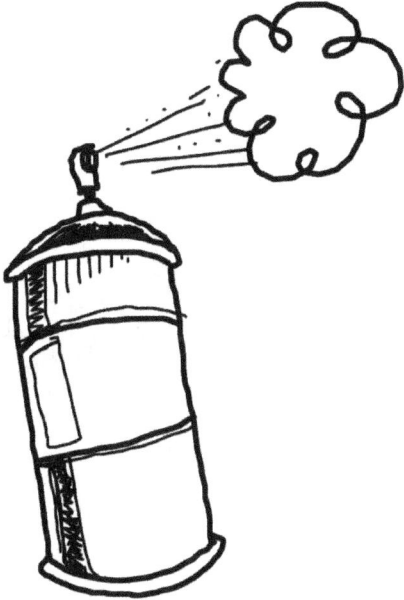

If you want to make deodorant or body spray, you can get the advantage of these recipes. Get the advantage of these recipes:

Recipe 31: DIY Deodorant

- Coconut oil: ½ cup

- Baking soda: ½ cup

- Essential oils of your choice: 40 to 60 drops

Directions:

Mix in coconut oil and baking soda in one bowl along with essential oils. Store this deodorant in a glass jar and use as per your needs.

Recipe 32: Citrus Body Spray

- 15 Drops Grapefruit EO

- 5 drops of Lavender EO

- 8 Ounces distilled Water

- 1 tablespoon Hazel

Directions:

In the first step, add vodka (if using) in one jar and put all the ingredients and shake them well. It will be good to secure this mixture in a dark bottle and put this bottle in one dark and cold place for almost seven days. You can rub it on your pulse points to enjoy the enduring fragrance.

Recipe 33: Comfort Your Body

- Distilled Water: 8 Ounces

- Hazel: 1 tablespoon

- Cinnamon leaf EO: 10 drops

- Sweet orange EO: 15 drops

Directions:

In the first step, add vodka (if using) in one jar and put all the ingredients and shake them well. It will be good to secure this mixture in a dark bottle and put this bottle in one dark and cold place for almost seven days. You can rub it on your pulse points to enjoy the enduring fragrance.

Recipe 34: Body Spray to Empower Your Brain

- Distilled Water: 8 Ounces

- Hazel: 1 tablespoon

- Rosemary oil: 5 drops

- Patchouli oil: 10 drops

- Peppermint oil: 10 drops

Directions:

In the first step, take one jar and put all the ingredients and shake them well. It will be good to secure this mixture in a dark bottle and put this bottle in one dark and cold place for almost seven days. You can rub it on your pulse points to enjoy the enduring fragrance.

Recipe 35: Jasmine Deodorant

- Distilled water: 1 tablespoon

- Vodka: 2 tablespoons

Jasmine blend

- Lavender: 5 drops

- Jasmine: 30 drops

- Vanilla: 5 drops

Directions:

In the first step, add vodka (if using) in one jar and put all the ingredients and shake them well. It will be good to secure this mixture in a dark bottle and put this bottle in one dark and cold place for almost seven days. You can rub it on your pulse points to enjoy the enduring fragrance.

Chapter 6 – Precautions to Use Essential Oil Perfumes

Essential oils and their perfumes are good for your skin. There are a few oils that should be used with special precautions. For your assistance, there is some guidance:

- There is no need to leave these oils in extreme temperatures, such as a freezer, hot cars, and near windows.

- Keep essential oils away from direct sunlight.

- Some essential oils can break down any plastic bottle; therefore, you shouldn't store them in plastic containers.

- It will be bad to keep the bottles of essential oils open because oxidation process can affect the potency of oil.

- There is no need to heat or boil your oils to allocate them aromatically. They can lose their therapeutic value.

- There is no need to use oils in the hot tub.

- Always use diluted essential oils because undiluted oils can irritate your skin.

- There is no reason to expose your skin to photosensitive oils before going out to the sun. After applying these oils to your skin, you should keep yourself away from the sun for almost 12 hours. All citrus oils are photosensitive oils.

- These oils are not good to put in your nose, eyes, and ears. If the essential oil accidently goes into your eyes, there is no need to use water to wash your eyes. It can increase your pain and chances of damage. You can use a carrier oil to draw any oil out of your eyes. You can also use a cotton cloth to clean oil from your eyes.

- If you are uncomfortable with any oil, you should avoid their use. There should search reliable oils by your sensitive skins and allergies.

- There is no need to give empty bottles of essential oils to your children to play. The residue of these oils will be there in the bottles; you should handle with care.

- You should be careful by using oils after and before bath and swimming. Sometimes, use of essential oils after taking a bath can cause clogging in open pores. The water may drive oil into your skin.

It is essential to keep these oils away from your pets and children. After coming out of tanning both, you should stay away from the sun for almost six hours after treatment. Essential oils have flammable qualities; hence, you should keep them away from fire, candles, gas cookers, matches, and cigarettes. You can test these oils on a small part of your skin to check allergies.

You can use fresh rose petals to diffuse them in base oils and mix essential oils in this diffused blend. There are various choices for you to make organic blends. It is time to get rid of ordinary perfumes full of chemicals. You can use recipes given in this book to make healthy combinations. These are equally good to send as a gift.

Organic perfumes require the use of essential oils, rose water and fruit extracts. You can buy your favorite ingredients from the market. Homemade perfumes are safe for your environment, and you can use them without any health problem. It is possible to make your dream fragrance and send it as a gift to your friends and impress them. If you want to send something unique, you can follow the recipes given in this book. There are lots of fragrances that you can use on different occasions. You can prepare a personalized fragrance for your wedding. It will be a good way to improve your overall health.

Conclusion

Replace all products with these homemade perfumes and body sprays. Nature has blessed us with amazing ingredients, and you can use all these ingredients to prepare your own fragrances. With children in your house, these perfumes and body sprays can be dangerous. This book is designed with 35 recipes that are perfect for you and your family. You can prepare your perfumes with the help of these recipes and improve your health and environment of your house.

There are recipes to make solid fragrances because the essential oils are available in the market. The perfumes in the market may have chemicals that are harmful to your skin. There is no need to spend your money on luxurious products because you can make organic perfumes at home. These perfumes are made of natural ingredients, and you may be able to save a good amount of money.

It is quite easy to make an organic fragrance, but you have to buy gloves, essential tools, containers and molds to make them. It is important to select a well-ventilated area so that you can protect yourself from the fumes and evaporation of some recipes. This book has recipes to make different kinds of fragrances protect your skin from allergies.